QUICK AND EASY FOOD

Joel Briggs

Contents

Chapter One

INTRODUCTION

A couple years ago, I learned that my wife had a problem I didn't know about. Celiac disease is an autoimmune disease that makes the person sensitive to gluten, a protein found in wheat, barley, and rye. When I looked into it, I found out it affects about half of the population and the symptoms are quite complex. I decided to write a book about the diet, and I started following the gluten-free diet. It has been a lifesaver for my wife and me, and the diet has changed our lives totally. It allowed us to become happy again, to find love and respect in our relationship, and to get back to being a family.

Celiac disease is an autoimmune disorder that affects up to 3 million Americans. Today, with gluten-free eating becoming more mainstream, celiac disease is considered a multisystem disorder, which means it can affect many systems of the body. Celiac disease is a digestive disorder. It is caused by gluten, a protein found in wheat, barley, and rye, which results in a flattening of the intestinal villi. It can be classified along with other autoimmune disorders as an autoinflammatory condition.

Although little research has been done in this area, the American Celiac Association believes that up to 10 percent of the population has gluten intolerance. This indicates that 30 million Americans experience gluten intolerance symptoms in their daily lives.

Some patients with celiac disease have a positive endoscopic biopsy, which shows the signs of damage to the villi in the small intestine. For other patients, however, the only way to tell whether they have celiac disease is through a diagnosis made by a physician or a doctor of internal medicine. When people say they have gluten intolerance, it is often difficult to tell if they are responding to gluten or if they have another illness that may be causing similar symptoms.

I often describe myself as a simple cook. I make bread when I'm feeling like baking, and I love to make a good cup of coffee. All of my family and friends know that my husband and I try to eat gluten-free, and I cook gluten-free whenever I can, because I know how difficult it is for my husband (who suffers from celiac disease) to find gluten-free foods. My first cookbook was about a family who follows a gluten-free diet, so it is always fun to come up with new recipes for gluten-free foods. I don't need to be lectured when it comes to what my

After she began a gluten-free diet, Isabeau didn't experience nearly the same problems as her mother experienced with wheat. For example, she was more than fine with her wheat pastas and sauces. She enjoyed cheese pizza for the first time. And her taste buds began to detect all sorts of flavors that they had previously overlooked.

I want to extend a heartfelt thank you, in part, because my five-year-old daughter, Isabeau, has celiac disease. It has been challenging finding gluten-free foods that meet her taste buds. I read your book, The Gluten-Free Diet, for the first time on a whim. My mom bought it for me at a health food store. The more I read, the more the book and recipes appealed to me. I wanted to bring some of your recipes to Isabeau. She was apprehensive at first, but I could tell by her smile that the dishes were getting approval. I have to say, Isabeau has such a beautiful smile, and this recipe for Cinnamon Rolls gave me a new appreciation for her. I now have to give Isabeau a bowl of chocolate ice cream. You have brought so much joy to our lives through your cookbook and your story.

Cassandra and Isis

In addition to a chapter of easy-going, feel-good foods, this book also contains recipes that are truly unique. Many of the dishes in these chapters were originally popular with celiacs and contain gluten-free ingredients. Many people don't realize the extent they have been exposed to gluten. Some dishes are easy to adapt, while others are very tricky. To adapt a dish for a gluten-free diet, be sure to find a substitute for the gluten source in the original recipe. Many of the dishes listed have gluten-free substitutions with the same flavor profile but in a gluten-free base.

In my first gluten-free cookbook, my primary goal was to teach readers how to cook in a simple, gluten-free way for people with either no cooking experience or limited cooking experience. Many of the same recipes from the first book are included in this cookbook, with many changes to make the dishes even more flexible and appealing to a wider range of gluten-free dieters who might enjoy different types of foods or who just want more choices. Quick-Fix Gluten Free also includes new recipes for those who may need gluten-free flour, baking mixes, or other gluten-free baking ingredients. A section on gluten-free flours

This cookbook includes more than 200 recipes, which take less than 30 minutes or, in many cases, less than 10 minutes to prepare. Recipes that take less than half an hour are listed on pages 24 and 25, with an extra ten minutes or more of time indicated. There are also some helpful tips and tricks for minimizing prep time, including a recipe for a gluten-free bread, which is easy to make and tastes great! This book is intended as a reference tool for your kitchen that will help you to prepare quick meals for yourself, your family, and even take out fast for a busy weeknight.

We've seen an increase in the quality, texture, and taste of gluten-free food products. In addition, numerous products have appeared on the market, giving gluten-free recipe ideas for every meal and every occasion. At the same time, all ingredients must be made gluten-free, and that means it is impossible to make them all. One loaf of bread may vary in taste and consistency from another. This cookbook was made from recipes available to the public on the market. This book offers gluten-free recipes and gluten-free baking ideas that can be prepared for any meal and any occasion.

In this book, you will discover what it means to make a quick meal for yourself. You will find recipes for delicious breakfasts and brunches, such as a Spinach, Bacon, and Cheddar Pie, and Cinnamon-Raisin French Toast, along with appetizers including Tangy Peanut Butter Chicken Skewers, Sharp Cheese Potato Croquettes, and Savory Swedish Meatballs. There is a salad section with dishes such a The Perfect Caesar Salad with Her

Here are some recipes that I shared in the first bread chapter to help you use bread more creatively. You will find recipes for Rosemary Garlic Baguettes, Grilled Pizza Crust, and Molasses Flax Sandwich Bread. There are others for the chapter about Tasty Comforts that provide international comfort food favorites, such as Plum Barbecued Baby Back Ribs, Golden Walnut Baked Stuffed Shrimp, and Turkey and Tart Apple Meat Loaf.

For those who are looking for a quick, easy snack, this recipe is for you! It includes all-natural sweet potato gnocchi and three-cheese penne with roasted garlic butter, peas, and bacon. If you've got time to spare, you can bake the dish with a delicious pudding with chocolate, banana, and espresso.

1 Peter H.R. Green and Rory Jones.

2 Dr. Stephen Wangen, Healthier Without Wheat (Seattle: Innate Health Publishing, 2009), 22–23.

Speed up your preparation time.

At the beginning, I always use the 'everything' method. But as life goes on, the kitchen has become messier and I have to "cook in a rush." I should probably spend more time to organize my kitchen, rather than "cook in a rush."

Kitchen Equipment

This book is easy to use with basic kitchen utensils. Some of the recipes call for special equipment, such as a hand mixer and food processor, but you will find many other recipes that do not require these expensive tools. In addition, a glass of wine will make some of the recipes go down easy and make cooking simple.

When I read about gluten free foods I thought "Now I'm sure gluten-free foods is for me." After reading this the thought came into my mind that I can have as many as I want. The gluten free foods that I was reading about, I can have as many as I want. These are just a few examples of signature breakfast items of which I have developed gluten-free versions for this chapter, to bring back to you what you thought might be gone forever.

When my wife and I sold our bakery, we thought about creating various healthy breakfast recipes. But, when we tried testing the recipes, we learned that our gluten-free flour blends weren't close to the traditional blends. We decided to go back in time and replicate some of the classic Sugar Shack recipes. Many times afterward, I would ask Angela if she missed some of those classic treats. So, I decided to go back in time, recreate these old recipes, and share some of our favorites with you. Our goal is to encourage you all to jump out of bed, and start your day out just right. Original: 1.1. Introduction 1.2. Basic terms 1.3. Background of the topic 2.1. Communication 2.2. Communication and culture 2.3. Global perspectives on communication 2.4. Cultural differences in communication 2.5. Gender differences in communication 2.6. Theore

Chapter Two

RECIPES

Belgian waffles

creates 6 to 8 servings

Whole-grain flaxseed meal gives these waffles a nutty flavor and a whole-grain appeal, making them just as chewy and delicious as the original ones without the use of eggs or baking powder. Top the waffles with fresh berries and you've just made a nutritious and delicious start to the

1 cup of tapioca flour

¼ cup flour.

¼ cup white rice flour

2 tablespoons of flaxseed

Two tablespoons of brown sugar

One teaspoon baking soda

½ teaspoon ground cinnamon

½ teaspoon salt

3 whole eggs

Make it with buttermilk

1 teaspoon vanilla bean paste

3 tablespoons unsalted butter

Maple syrup, for serving

A side of fresh strawberries, please

No blueberries, for serving

Whipped cream, for serving (optional)

Preheat a waffle iron.

In a medium bowl, combine the tapioca flour, corn flour (polenta), white rice flour (regular or superfine, whichever the original recipe calls for), flaxseed meal, brown sugar, baking soda, cinnamon, salt, and

In a big bowl, make an omelet. Beat together the eggs, buttermilk, vanilla, and melted butter.

Once you prepare the wet ingredients, gradually add the dry ingredients to the wet until the ingredients are well mixed. Set the batter aside.

Beat egg whites in bowl with an electric mixer until stiff peaks form. Use a spatula to fold egg whites into the batter until blended.

Put a tablespoon or two of nonstick cooking spray on the grids and then ladle the batter in. Cook the waffles for 2-3 minutes and then serve plain. If you don't like whipped cream, the waffles are delicious by themselves.

Buttermilk pancakes

Makes 4 servings

After my son was asked "What do you want for breakfast?" he always replied, "Pancakes!" Now, with this lighter and fluffier gluten-free version, everyone will want to make pancakes and sing their approval of the pancakes. Let the pancakes go away by adding items like dark chocolate chips, blueberries, butterscotch chips, bananas, or

¼ cup tapioca

1/4 cup corn flour

¼ cup all-purpose flour

One teaspoon baking powder

2 tablespoons flaxseed meal

A teaspoon granulated sugar

1 cup buttermilk

1 egg

1 tablespoon of vegetable oil

1 teaspoon vanilla paste

Serve maple syrup

In a bowl, stir together gluten-free flour, corn flour, rice flour, flaxseed meal, and sugar. Add salt and whisk to mix.

Combine the buttermilk, egg, oil, and vanilla in the bowl. Make sure they're well combined; add the ingredients together in a separate bowl.

Whisk the dry ingredients into the wet.

Pour 1/4 cup batter into a heavy nonstick skillet to make a golden crusted pancake.

Chef's note: You can add any of your favorite pancake mix-ins after you've made a pancake.

Cinnamon-raisin french toast

Ready in 4 minutes.

This recipe was created by autism support group members who wanted to find a quick, gluten-free and dairy-free food that was also yummy. The result was this cinnamon-dusted French toast, which was a crowd pleaser. The kids especially liked it.

A cup of milk or nondairy alternative

5 grams of sugar

¼ teaspoon salt

3 to 4 teaspoons of ground cinnamon

3 eggs

A tablespoon of butter, peanut butter, or other alternative.

Find 12 slices Udi's Cinnamon Raisin Bread

Chocolates for serving

Serve Maple Syrup.

In a medium bowl, whisk together the milk, granulated sugar, and salt. Whisk in the cinnamon and eggs.

Melt the butter for about 3 minutes

Dredge the bread in the egg mixture, covering both sides.

Allow the surplus egg to drip out of between the bread slices before placing them in the hot pan and cooking for just a minute on each side.

Slather the French toast with confectioners' sugar, keeping it warm if desired, and then serve with maple syrup.

Top-of-the-morning muffins

Makes 12

Bake time: 25 to 30 minutes

A mixture of walnuts, raisins, apple, carrot, coconut and applesauce makes this cake the best thing since sliced bread. My wife has a tendency to always top them with cream cheese or frosting, which she considers a great indul

½ cup of sorghum flour

One and a half cups brown rice flour

1 cup white rice flour

4 tablespoons tapioca flour

A teaspoon of xanthan gum

1 teaspoon baking soda

½ teaspoon salt

1 teaspoon honey plus ⅛ teaspoon cinnamon

¼ teaspoon ground ginger

Use ¼ teaspoon ground nutmeg in your batter

1 stick of butter at room temperature

½ cup plus ½ tablespoon granulated sugar

½ cup packed brown sugar

½ cup apples, ¼ cup oatmeal

2 whole eggs beaten

1 cup of shredded carrots

¼ cup walnuts

¼ cup shredded sweetened coconut

¼ cup raisins

Preheat the oven to 350 degrees.

Put the sorghum flour, rice flour, white rice flour, tapioca flour, xanthan gum, baking soda, and salt in a bowl and stir to mix. Add 1 teaspoon of the cinnamon, ginger, and nutmeg to the mixture.

Stir together in a mixing bowl: • 1/3 cup of butter, • ½ cup of granulated sugar, • ¼ cup of brown sugar, • 1 cup applesauce, • 1 egg, • 1 apple, diced, or 1 cup of carrots, ½ cup of finely chopped walnuts, and ¼ cup of coconut, • Add raisins and bake in muffin cups • With a teaspoon of cinnamon mixed in with 2 tablespoons of granulated sugar, sprinkle on top of baked muffins.

Very berry muffins

Makes 12

Cooking time: 25 to 30 minutes

These sweet and soft gluten-free muffins are a treat for any morning, served with a steaming cup of coffee, because they're that good!

½ cup of sorghum flour

½ cup brown rice flour

¾ cup white rice flour

1/4 cup tapioca flour

1/2 teaspoon baking soda

1 teaspoon xanthan gum

½ teaspoon of salt

6 tablespoons of butter at room temperature

1 ½ cups plus 1 tablespoon

½ cup brown sugar

½cup (250ml) milk

1 egg

One and a half cups of mixed fresh or frozen berries (raspberries, blueberries, and blackberries)

Preheat the oven to 350°F

In a large bowl, place sugar, sorghum flour, brown rice flour, white rice flour, baking powder, xanthan gum and salt. Mix well to blend all ingredients. A: Original sentence: The

Using an electric mixer, mix together the butter and the sugars until light and fluffy. Then add the milk and the egg, and beat until it gets creamy and frothy. Add the flour and mix to uniform texture. Fold in the berries and place the batter in muffin tins until two-thirds full. Top with sugar and bake for 25 to 30 minutes, until a toothpick inserted into the center of a muffin comes out clean.

The ultimate cookie that starts your day with healthy calories and protein

They're very useful

Baking time: around 15 minutes

When I was asked by a friend how to make oatmeal cookies without flour, I tried them. They were pretty good, so I tried them for breakfast. Now that I have perfected these flavorful cookies, I always have them for breakfast.

4½ cups gluten-free oatmeal

Put 1 teaspoon of baking soda in the bath to disinfect and sanitize.

½ flaxseed meal

1 cup natural peanut butter

Three tablespoons of butter, at room temperature

1 cup packed brown sugar.

¾ cup granulated sugar

1/4 cup honey

2 bananas, mashed

3 eggs, lightly beaten

1 teaspoon vanilla vanilla extract

¼ cup almonds, chopped

A   cup of tiny chocolate chips

About ½ teaspoon roasted unsalted sunflower seeds

Set the oven to 350°F.

Combine the oats, baking soda, and flaxseed meal in a medium bowl.

Using a hand mixer, combine the peanut butter, butter, brown sugar, granulated sugar, and honey in another bowl. Beat in the eggs and vanilla. Then slowly mix in the oat mixture, stopping periodically to stir. Stir in the almonds, chocolate chips and sunflower seeds until combined.

Drop tablespoons of dough two inches apart evenly on ungreased cookie sheets. Bake at 350 degrees for 12 to 14 minutes. The cookies should be golden brown and then cooled.

For an even healthier take on this cookie, substitute dried fruit such as apples, dates, or figs for the chocolate chips.

Glazed cinnamon rolls

Makes 12

1 Hour

Time to bake: 15 to 20 minutes

I firmly believe that once you taste these, you will never want to go back eating the old cinnamon roll. I came up with this version that is gluten-free, sweet and chewy. You will love these cinnamon rolls!

2/3 cup buttermilk

¼ cup apple or orange juice

¼ teaspoon granulated sugar

1 tablespoon of active dry yeast

1 ¼ cups tapioca flour

1 cup (100 g) wholemeal brown rice flour

¼ cup potato starch

¼ cup flaxseed powder

2½ teaspoons flax seed meal.

2 teaspoons of baking powder

¼ teaspoon

One-quarter teaspoon baking soda

A quarter of a teaspoon of ground cinnamon.

2 tablespoons of butter, melted

1 tablespoon vegetable oil

1 egg and 1 egg white

1 teaspoon vanilla extract

FILLING

½ cup packed brown sugar

¼ cup of granulated sugar

2 teaspoons ground cinnamon

4 tablespoons (½ stick) butter melted

¼ cup chopped walnuts is the ideal snack.

GLAZE

¾ cup of confectioners' sugar

1/2 tablespoon milk

½ teaspoon vanilla extract

Pour the buttermilk in a bowl and heat it until the temperature rises to 110 degrees. Add the sugar and the yeast, and mix. The yeast should be in the mixture and it should be warm. Set aside.

Prepare a large bowl by combining the ingredients. The dough will be sticky. Cover dough with a greased bowl and allow to rise for 1 hour, or until doubled in bulk.

Meanwhile, prepare the mixture of Grease the muffin tin and set aside.

Use 1 teaspoon of flour until the surface appears dry. Then, coat the exposed surface with melted butter. Place the butter-coated surface on top of another sheet of wax paper. Sprinkle the sugar filling evenly over the butter, followed by the walnuts. Place the bottom piece of wax paper onto the waxed paper surface and roll the dough away from you into a 15 by 10-inch rectangular shape. Once the dough is rolled, seal the edges of the dough and cut into 12 even slices 1/4 inch thick. Place the slices cut side down into the muffin tins. Cover with a clean dish towel and place in a warm spot to rise for 1 hour, until the dough reaches the top of the muffin tin.

A recipe for delicious cinnamon rolls includes confectioners' sugar, milk, and vanilla. The mixture is poured over a plate of just-warm cinnamon rolls. The glaze can be drizzled over the rolls to add a delicious extra flavor.

Sweet cheese crêpes with caramelized peaches and granola

Make it a meal

The scrumptious, caramel-coated, peach- and granola-filled crêpes were a perfect fit for the cover of this recipe book.

½ cup white flour

1/4 cup tapioca flour

¼ cup corn flour.

Put ½ teaspoon of xanthan gum in water.

2 teaspoons of sugar.

½ teaspoon salt

1 cup milk

A cup of water

3 eggs

2 sticks butter

1 teaspoon of vanilla

Sweet cheese filling (following recipe)

Peach Topping (recipe below)

¼ cup "Gone Completely Nuts" Granola

In a large mixing bowl, mix the all-purpose flour, cornstarch, tapioca flour, xanthan gum, sugar and salt thoroughly.

In a bowl, combine the milk, water, eggs, butter, vanilla, and flour. Mix well and add the fruit. Blend for 10 seconds. Pour the batter into a greased, 10-inch, two-piece, heavy cake pans and bake for 45 to 50 minutes

Spray a nonstick pan with nonstick cooking spray. Cook about 2 tablespoons of batter in the center of the pan, but do not spray the pan with nonstick cooking spray, swirl the pan to form a thin pancake, and cook for 50 to 60 seconds. Flip over with a spatula and cook until it is firm to the touch, about 10 to 15 seconds. Place the pancake on a sheet of wax paper to cool and continue making crêpes with the remaining

After having all the crêpes cooled, spread 1 to 1½ tablespoons of the cheese filling on half of each crêpe. Then fold the crêpe in half once and then again, so that it makes a triangular envelope. Place on a plate and continue to spread the filling on the other crêpes.

Put 1 tablespoon of the remaining butter in a large nonstick pan. Then add half of the crêpes, let them cook over medium heat for 1 to 2 minutes, flip them over and cook for another minute. Put the cooked crêpes on a platter, and cook the remaining crêpes in 1 tablespoon of butter.

To serve individual crêpes, prepare four to six. Sprinkle the crêpes with peach topping before topping them with a spoonful of granola.

To save space, prepare the unfilled crêpes in advance and stack them between layers of wax paper in resealable plastic bags. This is a very good shortcut. It will save you time, since you won't need to make each one fresh. # Here

Cheesecake

1 bowl of cottage cheese, room temperature

2 tablespoons of brown sugar

½ teaspoon of cinnamon

¾ teaspoon ground nutmeg

Using an electric mixer with a paddle, beat together the cream cheese, brown sugar, and cinnamon for two minutes.

Peach topping

1 teaspoon butter

The weight of 1 lb. frozen sliced peaches, thawed and cut in half

Two tablespoons of brown sugar

¼ teaspoon ground cinnamon

Heat one tablespoon of butter in an oversized skillet. Then add the peaches to it, add the brown sugar and cinnamon and watch the peaches cook for five minutes.

Spinach, bacon, and cheddar pie

Makes 1 (9-inch) pie

Bake time: 50 to 55 minutes

This egg pie is similar to quiche but is lighter and fluffier. Its classic savory combination of bacon, cheese, and fresh baby spinach baked into an irresistible crust guarantees it will be an Easter brunch favorite. The tutorial on this page will show you how to make a gluten-free crust.

Cheddar cheese pie

1 cup of regular whole wheat flour

1 cup tapioca flour

1 tablespoon of granulated sugar

Two-tablespoon baking soda

½ teaspoon xanthan gum

½ teaspoon sodium

¼ cup of vegetable shortening

¼ cup of shredded cheddar or Swiss cheese

4 tablespoons (½ stick) butter (450 g, or 1 lb)

½ cups milk a

FILLING

1 cup packed baby spinach

Half a pound of bacon, cooked until crispy

2 scrambled eggs, 1 cheese and 3 fried eggs

You can use a one-and-a-half cups of light cream or half-and-half

½ cup grated sharp cheddar or Swiss cheese

Add a pinch of salt

Add a pinch of freshly ground black pepper

To make the crust: Beat the shortening and cheese together in a medium bowl. Add the white rice flour, tapioca flour, sugar, baking soda, xanthan gum, and salt, and continue to mix these together. Add the shredded

For pastry, use a pastry blender to mix shortening and butter. It is important to use a food processor for this step. If using a food processor instead, cut fat into butter before adding milk. Also, use your hands to mix the dough instead.

Place the pastry dough on a countertop or cutting board. Peel off the wax paper. Invert and place the pie plate on top to cover the dough. Press and trim the edges with a knife. Fold a corner over another to form a cup and crimp the edges using your fingers. --- Original: I find the perfect word for a person who will listen to all sides of a discussion and look for the best resolution, but still has a stubborn, haughty and self-centered personality. That's a perfect word, and it has a lot of meaning. Paraphrase: This person has an

Preheat the oven to 350 degrees.

To fill the pie: Top the spinach and bacon with a layer of spinach and bacon.

Preheat the oven to 375 degrees Fahrenheit. Whisk the eggs, cream, cheese, salt, and pepper together in a large bowl. Cover the bottom of a pie crust with the spinach and bacon. Bake for

50 to 55 minutes, until a knife inserted in the center comes out clean.

Blueberry and cream cheese strata

Makes approximately 6 to 8 servings.

Your baking time is one hour

In this recipe, you'll be baking bread and cream cheese, then drizzling it with maple syrup before serving.

2 (eight-ounce) loaves Udi's White Sandwich or whole grain bread and

Six ounces of cream cheese, cubed

1 cup (6 ounces) fresh or drained frozen blueberries

8 eggs

1 cup whole milk or heavy whipping cream

¼ cup maple syrup, plus more for drizzling

4 tablespoons (½ stick) butter, melted

½ teaspoon of vanilla

A pinch of cinnamon works great

½ teaspoon grated nutmeg

A pinch of dusting sugar

Place half of the bread cubes in an 11 x 7 (inch) baking dish, followed by the cream cheese cubes and the blueberries. Add the remaining bread cubes on top of the blueberries.

Whisk together the eggs, milk,   cup of the syrup, melted butter, vanilla, cinnamon, and nutmeg in a medium bowl. Combine the bread and the egg mixture and cover with aluminum foil and refrigerate for 2 hours.

Prepare a large baking sheet by lining it with a piece of parchment paper. To this, pour the mixture of chocolate chips and granulated sugar. Mix the two and bake for 30 minutes. Once the baketime is over, pull out the foil and bake for another 25 to 30 minutes, until the center is set and the edges are golden brown. Let it

"gone nuts" without losing the original word</

Makes 1½ pounds

Time to bake: 1 hour

This granola is nutty, honey-sweet, and full of delicious cranberries that give it a tart flavor as well as a healthy dose of antioxidants. It is also a good snack for watching movies.

1/4 cup of maple syrup

2 tablespoons of honey

1 tablespoon vegetable oil

3/4 cup unsweetened gluten-free oats

¼ cup chopped walnuts.

1 cup chopped pecans

½ cup unsalted, blanched, skinless almonds

½ cup lightly packed shredded coconut

¼ cup of brown sugar

½ teaspoon is the correct amount of salt

Add 1 cup dried cranberries or cherries into your diet

½ cup raisins (optional)

Preheat the oven to 250°F, and grease a baking sheet.

In a small bowl combine the liquid maple syrup, honey, and vegetable oil. Add the oats, walnuts, pecans, almonds, coconut, brown sugar, and salt and mix with an electric mixer until thoroughly combined.

Preheat the oven to 350° F. Arrange the bread ingredients in the baking pan in an even layer, and bake for 1 hour. Stir every 20 minutes and then allow to cool completely on the pan. When completely cool, add the dried cranberries and raisins, and store in an airtight container or resealable.

Grilled pineapple and apples with cinnamon on a skewer

4 servings at a time

Marinating time: 1 to 3 hours

It's the perfect way to get more of your daily requirement of fruit. These slices of pineapple, nectarines, plums, and peaches are drizzled with vanilla, nutmeg, cinnamon, and maple syrup.

½ teaspoon maple syrup

1 tsp vanilla extract

¼ teaspoon ground nutmeg

Cinnamon tea can help you lose fat.

2 firm peaches, halved and pitted

A firm plum, halved, and pitted

2 firm nectarines, cut in half and pitted

1 cup pineapple chunks

4 wooden skewers, soaked in water for 20 minutes

1 pint of vanilla ice cream

To make this dessert, place the maple syrup, vanilla, cinnamon, nutmeg, and 2 cups of chopped apples in a medium bowl. Mix well. Set the fruit mixture aside for a few hours or overnight. Add the remaining cup of chopped apples to the fruit mixture, then toss to coat. Alternate the type of apple you use. Place the fruit skewers on the grill. Grill about 2 to 3 minutes per side until heated through and caramelized. Be sure to give the skewers a gentle turn to avoid burning the sides

Maple-drizzled fruits with toasted coconut

Makes 4 servings

Bake time: 1 hour

As an alternative to the ordinary morning banana, this pineapple, cantaloupe, honeydew, and grape salad is much healthier, light, and nutritious. Even if you only have a few minutes, you should enjoy this wonderful summer salad.

Yogurt is an amazing snack

A tablespoon of maple syrup.

½ cup pineapple cubes

½ cup grapes with skins

½ cup cantaloupe cubes

½ cup honeydew juice cubes.

1 tablespoon finely chopped fresh mint is all you need.

4 Tablespoons of shredded coconut, toasted

Whisk together the yogurt and juice and set aside.

Pour the salad ingredients into a large bowl. Mix them well.

Divide the fruit into four martini glasses with a dollop of yogurt and sprinkle some toasted coconut on top.

Appetizers, often served with a glass of wine, are typically tasty, flavorful, and sometimes teasing. However, what goes with appetizers can be as important as the food itself. Our friends Denise and Mike find a great variety of appetizers and order a number of different tasty dishes during meals. Together, the two of them will split three or four appetizers in lieu of a less-stuffed entrée, which allows them to sample a large variety of

As Angela and I have gotten older, our entertainment and entertaining are better than ever. We love the opportunity to offer our guests such an extraordinary appetizer for their upcoming meal. Over the years, they have mentioned how much they appreciate being able to munch on the unique dishes while socializing before the main course.

For celiacs, cheese and gluten-free crackers are a pre-meal mainstay. At this party, I'd set up appetizer stations offering Savory Swedish Meatballs—or a Cheesy Crab, Spinach and Artichoke Dip, for the guests who crave traditional pub appetizers.

Grilled Feta and Zucchini Medallions with Lemon-Garlic Yogurt Sauce

Yields 4~6 servings

This vegetarian delight is prepared by combining lots of summer squash, a bit of feta cheese, and a small amount of rice flour

2 small zucchini (about ½ pound)

Two medium yellow squash (about a pound)

1 cup gluten-free bread crumbs

3/4 cup crumbled feta cheese (about 4 ounces)

¼ cup of minced Vidalia or other sweet onion

2 tablespoons white rice flour

1 tablespoon finely chopped fresh dill

1/5 teaspoon salt

Add grated cheese to your pasta, risotto, or other pasta dishes

Beat a single egg

2 Tbsp or more unsalted butter or more as needed

2 tablespoons of vegetable oil and more as needed

Lemony Lamb's Liver (recipe follows)

Grate the zucchini and squash into a medium bowl.

Blend the mixture and transfer to a strainer. The result was a thick slurry. I transferred this back to the dried bowl, then pressed it down with my hand, to squeeze out

Take the brown rice flour, cheese, onion, dill, salt and pepper.

Form and shape the batter into 2-inch patties.

In a small skillet, put the butter and oil.

Cook the burgers for 3 to 4 minutes per side, adding more butter and oil when needed.

Lay the burgers on a platter with a dollop of the sauce on each.

Lemon garlic yogurt sauce

Choose Greek yogurt

2 cloves garlic, finely chopped

One teaspoon freshly squeezed lemon juice

⅛ teaspoon cayenne, a little spice

Combine all the ingredients together in a small food processor and blend until completely combined. Refrigerate until needed. When it's needed, whisk or beat it until it's fluffy.

Dried apricots and gorgonzola cheese

Makes two dozen

A full range of flavors: sweet, bitter, salty, rich, and smoky, and a hint of nuttiness.

24 Medjool dates

24 unsalted roasted almonds

Two ounces of goat cheese

12 strips bacon, halved crosswise.

Preheat your oven to 400°F and lightly grease a baking pan.

Grate an almond on top of dates, stuff dates with goat cheese, and wrap each date tightly in bacon. Place the date on the baking pan seam side down and grill or broil until the bacon is crispy, about 10 minutes. After it's cooked, remove from the oven, allow them to cool, and serve at room temperature.

Savory Swedish meatballs.

Can eat 30 to 40 pounds of food each day.

All over the world, this favorite food item originated in Sweden and now comes a gluten-free version from a small town in Connecticut. It's a blend of small pieces of gluten-free bread kneaded into ground pork and then topped with red currant jelly. You won't care whether or not the country it came from.

3 pieces of Udi's White Bread, cut into small pieces

½ cup half-and-half

2 tablespoons plus 1 tablespoon unsalted Butter.

½ cup minced onion

One pound ground beef

One pound ground meat

2 eggs, beaten

1/2 teaspoon kosher salt

Take 1/2 teaspoon of ground allspice.

¼ teaspoon freshly ground pepper.

¼ teaspoon brown mustard

Put ground nutmeg into your body

Two tablespoons of white rice flour

2 cups of beef broth

¼ cup sour cream

2 tablespoons of red-currant jelly

In a small bowl, combine the bread and half-and-half and set aside.

In the medium skillet over medium heat, melt 2 tablespoons of butter. Add the onions and cook, stirring occasionally, for 3 to 4 minutes, until tender.

To make the barbecue sauce, beat together the cranberries, vinegar, brown sugar, and garlic in a large bowl. Stir in the mayonnaise, tomato paste, pepper, and mustard until well blended.

Use a measuring cup to scoop the ground meat into a meat-freezing bag and pat it to form 1-inch balls.

Heat the remaining 2 tablespoons of the butter in medium-sized skillet and add the meatballs to the pan. Cook the meatballs over medium heat without crowding in the pan, and continue to cook for about 10 minutes or until slightly golden and cooked through. Transfer the cooked meatballs to a baking dish and keep warm in a warm oven.

After all the meatballs are completely cooked on the stove, add the white rice flour and whisk to blend the flour with the drippings on the stove. Slowly add the beef broth and continue whisking until the sauce becomes thick and smooth, 3 to 4 minutes. Whisk in the sour cream and jelly and simmer until the sauce is thick and creamy, so that it coats the back of a spoon.

Fill a serving dish with the meatballs and gravy, and serve.

Blue cheese and spinach–stuffed mushrooms

Makes 40

These stuffed mushrooms are a festive must-have around the home, and people have even reported sneakily popping one right after another.

1½ cups of hot gluten-free chicken broth

1½ cups (about 6 ounces) Aleia's Savory Stuffing Mix

1. (10-ounce) packet thawed and drained spinach

Make dinner out of around 40 medium mushrooms.

2 teaspoons butter

2 cloves of garlic, minced

¼ ounce blue cheese

A ½ cup cup finely grated Parmesan cheese

Preheat the oven to 400°F and preheat an oven.

Add all of the ingredients to the large bowl and, using a fork, mix everything until it's all well-blended.

Remove the stems from the mushrooms and dice.

Melt the butter in a skillet over medium-high heat. Add the mushroom stems and garlic and cook until tender, about 5 minutes. Add to stuffing mixture, along with the blue cheese and Parmesan, and mix to incorporate.

Take the mixture and spoon it into the mushroom caps. Place the mushrooms on baking pan and bake them for about 15 minutes. Make sure that the liquid has been absorbed, and that the mushrooms are done.

It is very important that you read labels properly to avoid consuming breaded/baked/topped mushrooms. They can be made one day ahead and refrigerated for a day.

Garlic herbed cheese spread

Makes roughly 1½ cups

"It's important to find a quick, easy, and delicious appetizer that can be enjoyed by all," says James McBride. James helps restaurants by creating recipes and recipes that are accessible to everyone.

2 teaspoons of garlic.

¼ teaspoon salt (no, not a typo)

8 tablespoons (1 stick) butter, at room temperature

A room-temperature package of cream cheese

½ teaspoon dried oregano

⅛ teaspoon dried thyme leaves

⅛ teaspoon dried marjoram leaves

½ teaspoon dried dill

1/16 teaspoon freshly ground black pepper

Chop the garlic finely. Sprinkle with salt. Rub the garlic paste to a paste with a knife.

Sift together the butter, Neufchâtel cheese, garlic paste, and other spices.

For a cheese that is best served chilled, put the cheese in an apparent, and let it sit out for a few minutes. Remove when you're ready, and serve.

Sweet and spicy Korean fried chicken.

Makes 6 servings

Marinating time: overnight

One family reunion in New Jersey had a potluck dinner, and four different people started cooking the chicken wings. But these were the first that people tried, and they were the only ones left to serve.

1 cup of milk

Two tablespoons of granulated sugar

Two teaspoons of salt

1/2 teaspoon freshly ground black pepper

1/2 teaspoon ground ginger

3 pounds of chicken wings

1¾ cup white rice flour

¼ cup potato starch

I usually use one and a half tablespoons curry powder.

3 tablespoons of chopped sweet onion

Use 1 tablespoon olive oil

One-third cup tomatoes with one cup of tomato sauce.

¼ cup sweet chili sauce

½ cup water

1 tablespoon gluten-free Worcestershire sauce

Fat for deep frying

2 green onions, finely chopped

The milk is mixed with the sugar and salt and some pepper, and it is whisked in a large bowl. This step is repeated to bring out the flavor of the milk. This is done after the wings have been marinated for several hours in the refrigerator

In a medium bowl, whisk together the water, rice flour, and potato starch. Set aside.

In a medium saucepan, heat the olive oil over medium heat. Add the onion and cook until softened. Add the tomato sauce, chili sauce, water and Worcestershire sauce, and simmer until the sauce begins to thicken, about 5 minutes; set aside.

In a large frying pan, heat 2 inches of vegetable oil until it gets to 350 degrees. While the oil heats up, pat the wings dry with a paper towel.

Put 6 to 8 wings at a time into the seasoned flour and then add them to a hot oil to fry. Take them out once they turn light brown. To make sure the wings aren't sticking together, shake some flour on them.

To a well-to-do couple's home, they added a new, smaller kitchen. And there are plans underway to renovate the family's kitchen again. However, the couple has decided that only a well-to-do couple should have a kitchen of this kind, the man said.

Sesame-coconut onion rings with orange marmalade dipping sauce

Makes two servings:

The original chef developed the light batter that holds the onions together while allowing the ring to retain a crisp texture and the flavors of the other ingredients.

¾ cup white rice flour

¼ cup almond flour 1. In each of the new sentences you are creating, select a word at the end of the sentence that you

1/3 cup of shredded coconut with 1/3 cup of brown sugar.

2 tablespoons of sesame seeds

Use 1 teaspoon salt.

¼ teaspoon of cayenne

2 eggs in the morning

¾ cup gluten-free beer

Peanut oil, for deep frying

Two sweet, yellow onions, cut into ½-inch rings

Orange Marmalade Dipping Sauce

Add the egg yolks, beer, sesame seeds, and spices to a medium bowl. Whisk until a smooth batter forms.

To make a very light batter, start with a breadcrumb mixture, then add just enough flour to make the batter a little thicker than cake batter. This step is important so the batter does not stick to the onions.

Make a delicious orange marmalade dipping sauce

1 cup orange marmalade

¼ cup of Dijon mustard

¼ cup of honey

Whisk together the orange marmalade, Dijon mustard, and honey,

Grilled vegetable platter

Makes 6 to 8 servings

This grilled vegetable salad is a common dish in Europe but has received very little attention here in the United States. It is the perfect platter to make for a vegetarian entrée or appetizer. You can also turn it into a meal for nonvegetarians by adding meat or prosciutto.

1 cup extra-virgin olive oil, plus extra for drizzling

Four cloves of garlic, peeled

3 fresh sprigs rosemary, chopped

Kosher salt and a freshly ground black

A small amount of sun-dried tomatoes

Two zucchini, cut lengthwise into ½ in slices

2 large yellow squash. Cut lengthwise into ½-inch slices.

1 medium eggplant, cut into ½-inch slices

2 large portobello mushrooms, stems removed

2 medium red onions, cut into ½ -inch thick slices

12 asparagus spears that have been trimmed

3 Italian-style frying peppers

1 bulb fennel, cut into quarters

Cut the lemon into thin slices.

1 (6-ounce) jar of marinated artichokes, drained

A cup of kalamata olives

6 fresh basil leaves and slivered

Balsamic vinegar, for drizzling

Turn on the grill medium/low.

In a small saucepan, heat the olive oil, garlic, rosemary, salt and pepper. Once the mixture is hot, let cool. Put the sun-dried tomatoes in a glass container and cover with the warm liquid. Refrigerate for about 10 minutes and drain.

Brush a heavy skillet, a cast-iron grill, or a metal grill pan with olive oil. Season the grill by brushing the grill surface with oil. Season the vegetables such that they are lightly brushed with olive oil. Sauté the vegetables over the grill for 4 to 5 minutes per side, just until slightly charred on the edges and tender. Remove the peppers from the grill, remove the stems and

Arrange vegetables and sun-dried tomatoes on a plate. Sprinkle with fresh basil leaves and season with salt and pepper. Garnish with a few grilled lemon slices and drizzle with extra-virgin olive oil and white balsamic vinegar.

Tangy peanut butter chicken skewers

Make 4 to 6 servings

Peanut butter and chicken skewers have been a popular snack in the United States for decades. This appetizer involves combining peanut butter and brown sugar, along with spices such as cayenne pepper and cinnamon, and then using an oven to bake the skewers and form a crispy coating. This appetizer is fun

2 pounds boneless, skinless chicken breasts, cut into 1-inch strips

Wooden skewers are soaked in water for 20 minutes

Make sure to use salt and pepper

½ cup peanut butter.

1/4 cup gluten-free chicken broth

1½ cups of water

¼ cup gluten-free miso

2 garlic cloves minced

Add 2 tablespoons freshly squeezed lime juice

2 tablespoons of brown sugar

¼ teaspoon ground ginger

⅛ teaspoon cayenne pepper

1 tablespoon chopped fresh cilantro

Preheat your grill at medium-high heat.

Make a skewer from the chicken. Slide the lemon and pepper onto the chicken, and sprinkle the chicken with salt and pepper. Cover the rest of the plate with the chicken.

In a medium saucepan over medium-high heat, combine the peanut butter, chicken broth, water, soy sauce, garlic, lime juice, brown sugar, ginger, and cayenne. Cook, stirring, until smooth and hot; set aside.

To prepare the chicken skewers, place the chicken pieces on the preheated grill. Brush generously with peanut butter sauce and cook for about 3 minutes on one side, then turn the chicken pieces and brush the other side with peanut butter sauce. Continue to grill, brushing on more sauces, until the chicken is cooked through, about 3 to 4 minutes. Serve with grilled pineapple.

Rice balls with cheese

Makes 24

These are an Italian treat—rice balls filled with cheese that have been breaded and deep fried.

2 cups gluten-free chicken broth

1 cup white rice

¼ cup finely grated Parmesan cheese

2 tablespoons chopped parsley

½ teaspoon of garlic powder

½ tsp freshly ground black pepper

2 eggs, as you would have them

½ cup gluten-free flour

The equivalent weight of about 2 ounces cheese (such as mozzarella, provolone, or Monterey Jack), cut into 24 cubes.

Vegetable oil for deep frying and oil

Put your broth in a large saucepan with high heat, then add in your rice, cover, lower heat, and simmer for 20 to 25 minutes, until all the water is absorbed.

Transfer the rice from an individual serving bowl to a large bowl. Stir the rice in the bowl with a fork or wooden spoon, and then stir in the Parmesan cheese, parsley, garlic powder, and pepper. Allow the rice to cool slightly and

In a separate bowl, beat the egg whites to froth.

Put the bread crumbs in a third bowl.

Combine one tablespoon of dry rice blend in the palm of your hand with one cube of cheese and form into a rice ball. Continue rolling the rice and cheese balls in the egg whites and bread crumbs until all of the rice balls are coated. Place the rice-cheese balls on a platter as you roll them in the egg whites and bread crumbs.

To make risotto, you need a large stock pot, lots of vegetables and rice, and a deep-fat thermometer. Heat three inches of oil until a deep-fat thermometer reading is 360°F. This will be the temperature of the oil when you add the risotti to the oil. Gently lower the rice balls into the hot oil and cook for about 1 to 2 minutes.

Spinach Parmesan Bites with a Honey Mustard Dipping Sauce

Makes 3 dozen

This savory stuffing mix by Aleia's is not only perfect because it holds the ingredients together perfectly, it also has a unique flavor that combines perfectly with the honey mustard dipping sauce.

¼ teaspoon Dijon mustard

Half of the sugar

2 (10-ounce) packages frozen chopped spinach, thawed and squeezed dry

A mixture of Aleia's sausage crumbles and herbs.

One cup freshly grated Parmesan cheese

8 tablespoons, solid butter or margarine

4 green onions with finely chopped leaves It shouldn't make a difference because you have the same title that's why you still receive the same salary

3 eggs, beaten

Use ¼ teaspoon of garlic powder.

Combine the honey and Dijon mustard in a small bowl, and set aside until needed.

In a large bowl combine together spinach, the stuffing mix tablespoon Parmesan cheese, a tablespoon of melted butter, green onions, an egg, and garlic powder; shape into 1-inch balls. Place balls on a platter covered with plastic wrap and place in the refrigerator overnight.

Preheat the oven at 350°F. Place a baking sheet in the oven.

First, put the spinach bites on a pan and bake them on an internal temperature of approximately 160 degrees Fahrenheit for 15 to 20 minutes, until golden brown. Serve them with a honey mustard sauce.

Sharp cheddar potato fried croquettes

The recipe makes a dozen

Cheese and potato croquettes, with a crispy exterior and a soft, creamy center—a cross between mashed potato and French fries.

A jug of water

¼ cup plus 1 teaspoon milk

1 big container of Betty Crocker's Potato Buds.

¼ c of finely grated cheese plus 1 tablespoon.

¼ teaspoon salt

¼ teaspoon freshly ground pepper

2 ounces of sharp cheddar cheese, cut into ½-inch cubes.

¼ cup oatmeal plus ¼ cup rice flour

1 egg

  cup gluten-free bread crumbs

Palm oil, for deep frying

In a medium saucepan, take one and a third of cups of water and a third cup of milk to a boil.

Leave the pan off the heat and stir in the stiff instant mashed potatoes.

Stir in ¼ cup of the Parmesan cheese, the salt, and the pepper.

Cut the tubuor dough in half.

Using a teaspoon, form potatoes into golf-ball-sized patties then wrap with cheese. Press cheese into the center of the patties.

Pour the flour in a bowl. Mix an egg and some milk.

Combine some bread crumbs and Parmesan cheese in a shallow dish.

Roll the potato balls in the flour, dip them in the egg mixture, and then coat them in bread crumbs.

Fill a saucepan halfway with vegetable oil and heat over medium-high heat, up to a temperature of 360°F degrees.

Bake the potato croquettes for ~2 to 3 minutes, until golden brown. Serve warm.

Sour cream, avocado, and grilled corn

Makes about 8 or 10 servings

Take your time to bake.

"High in calories, low on fat and has less than five grams of sugar, this dip is one of the best low-carbohydrate dips on the market," says Travis Diggs, owner of T-Town Chips.

1 (14oz) can artichoke hearts, quartered

1 (10-ounce) package frozen spinach, squeezed dry

1 (8-ounce) can of crabmeat

1 (8-ounce) package cream cheese, at room temperature

½ cup mayonnaise mixed into milk.

Make one cup of sour cream

½ cup shredded Cheddar cheese

½ cup shredded Monterey Jack cheese

3/4 cup plus 2 tablespoons finely grated Parmesan cheese

1 tablespoon Creole or stone-ground mustard

Add 1 teaspoon gluten-free Worcestershire sauce to the recipe.

½ teaspoon kosher salt

½ teaspoon celery seed

½ teaspoon cayenne

An egg yolk.

Bags of chips to serve

Prepare the oven to 350°F and grease a 12 by 8-inch casserole dish.

Beat together the artichoke hearts, spinach, crab, cream cheese, mayonnaise, sour cream, Jack cheese, Monterey Jack, ½ cup of Parmesan, Worcestershire sauce, kosher salt, cayenne, and egg yolk with an electric mixer with the paddle attachment

Pour the crab mixture into the prepared casserole dish, sprinkle evenly with the remainder of the Parmesan cheese, and cook over medium-high heat until the top becomes golden brown, and the center becomes hot, 30 minutes. Serve warm with tortilla chips.

Making salad dressing at home is usually more economical than buying a prepared.

I admit that my wife is more of a salad lover than I am. She can happily settle for a big bowl with all of her vegetables without any dressing. She does not like the dressings. When she does her salad, it is usually a bowl of greens with some sort of dressing, or maybe a chicken or vegetable sauce, etc. She does not like to look at an enormous bowl of salad. In her view, a salad is just a big bowl of food with no dressing. It can be made with an oil and vinegar or lemon juice; an oil and wine vinegar,

My goal for making a nutritious fresh salad is to make sure that all of the ingredients are fresh and ready to be used. Many people think that salads only contain ingredients that can be easily brought to the table: vegetables which can be prepared quickly or canned, potato chips, and canned chicken or tuna. On the contrary, I make sure that ingredients that are good for salad such as greens, vegetables, and avocados are fresh. No more than 2 to 3 hours before you plan to serve, I wash the ingredients thoroughly and then lay them out on a sheet pan in an area that is cool and dry. I use a salad spinner to separate the water so that I can drain what I don't need and the excess water will flow off when the greens are served.

There are three rules to assembling a salad. First, the greens must be cold, crisp, and crunchy. Usually, I'll place my washed and dried greens in a glass bowl, cover them with a clean dish towel, then place them in the back of the refrigerator where the temperature is coldest. Second, you must make a dressing that

Add the dressing just enough to lightly mix together the ingredients of the salad.

After I saw all those new people at the party, I became worried that I wasn't making any contribution. So to change things up, I decided to help plan the party and make a fun and creative salad! At the top you will find a salad cheat sheet that can be used to create salads that go beyond the basic lettuce and tomatoes. So, I hope you'll enjoy preparing and devouring them

This is a sample of some of the ingredients you can include on your salad. Try making a salad with some of your favorite ingredients, make your own unique and delicious salad, and then top the salad with an ingredient from this chapter.

Lettuce greens

"Iceberg" has a very long shelf life and a very mild flavor; they are practically calorie free.

Romaine: Crisp lettuce with a mild, smooth, and crispy texture that blends well with salad dressings. It is the lettuce of choice in a Caesar salad.

Buttered, Boston or Bibb lettuces: Lettuces with a gentle texture and mild flavor.

Green leaf or red leaf lettuce: It's not clear whether red leaf is actually greener than green. Both have a mild and delicate flavour, can be bought in huge bunches, and last longer in the crisper.

If you want to have energy and stay healthy, a great food choice would be spinach. This dark and leafy green has a uniqueness to it, has a rich flavor and has a lot of nutritional

Arugula: A peppery lettuce that tastes great eaten with other, milder greens.

Piquant: With a sharp flavor and high acidity

Romaine is: A crunchy green that needs to be blended with milder greens.

Mesclun, which is most definitely a catchall term, refers to a blend of other greens, such as arugula, watercress, mizuna, mustard greens, and sorrel.

Vinaigrette with honey and balsamic vinegar

You can make ¾ cup of batter

This light salad dressing is known for adding flavor and fun to any bowl of lettuce with fruit. I found that a fun and unique salad sauce at my barbeque and dinner parties.

A generous ¼ cup of balsamic and

1 tablespoon plus 1 teaspoon Dijon mustard

About 1 tablespoon of honey

¼ teaspoon salt

Pepper, a quarter teaspoon<|endoftext|>

2 tablespoons extra virgin olive oil

In a big bowl, combine the vinegar, mustard, honey, salt and pepper.

Stir in the oil, whisking constantly, until the dressing is emulsified.

Store in an airtight container in the refrigerator.

In the variation, add 1 clove garlic, minced or ¼ teaspoon garlic powder

Add 1 teaspoon dried oregano or Italian seasoning.

Buttermilk Ranch Dressing [

Makes one cup

The taste of your store-bought salad dressing is stale. The store-bought salad dressings also have high fat, low nutrition, and no nutritional value in them. Making your own salad dressing will change your way of shopping for vegetables.

2 oz buttermilk

¼ cup of mayonnaise

¼ cup sour cream

Chop 2 teaspoons of minced onion.

½ teaspoon freshly squeezed lemon juice

   teaspoon dry mustard

Add one-fourth teaspoon of garlic powder

One tablespoon finely chopped fresh parsley.

¼ teaspoon finely chopped fresh chives

¼ teaspoon of dried dill, or 1 -¼ teaspoon of chopped fresh

1/4 teaspoon salt

1/8 of a teaspoon freshly ground black pepper

Chill (optional) <|endoftext|>

In a medium bowl, whisk together all the ingredients. Cover and refrigerate for up to 1 week.

Hearty Blue Cheese Dressing

Makes 1 and 1/3 cups

If you have never had creamy, tangy homemade blue cheese dressing, you're missing out. It's very easy to make this dressing with only six ingredients and it's great on salads. If you're at the Super Bowl this year, slather the stuff on your Buffalo wings.

½ cup sour cream

½ cup mayonnaise

1/4 cup blue cheese, crumbled

2 tablespoons of plain, sifted buttermilk

Squeeze two tablespoons of organic lemon juice in one cup of water.

1/2 teaspoon finely chopped green onion.

¼ teaspoon salt

½ teaspoon freshly ground black pepper

In a medium bowl, cream all the ingredients. Place in a closed container and refrigerate for up to 1 week.

Chef's note: Blue cheese makers sometimes use breads that are made with wheat as the starting ingredient. So make sure you read the the labels on the package of cheese you buy.

French dressing

Makes enough for one cup

No more chemicals or stabilizers to gum up your salad dressing or let your veggies and greens dry out. This low-fat dressing is light and delicious, just like the French dressing.

½ cup extra-virgin olive oil

½ cup lemon juice + ¼ cup of apple cider vinegar + ¼ cup of water

6 tablespoons granulated sugar

1/4 teaspoon paprika

1 teaspoon Worcestershire sauce

Garlic will help build immunity

  teaspoon freshly ground black pepper

Two teaspoons Dijon mustard

1 dash of minced onion

In a medium bowl, whisk together the oil, vinegar, and sugar. Then sprinkle each side of the bread with paprika, Worcestershire sauce, black pepper, and garlic powder.

Put the Dijon mustard in a separate bowl, then slowly add the oil mixture, whisking constantly until the mixture is well blended. Stir in the onion and store in an airtight container. These are great with a simple sandwich.

Garlic caesar dressing

Makes enough for 1 cup

"This is a classic dish with a creamy sauce." It's a dish rich with creamy sauce and it's The perfect Caesar Salad.

3 cloves raw garlic

It may be a quarter cup

Two tablespoons of finely grated Parmesan cheese

Add a squeeze of lemon

1 tablespoon gluten-free Worcestershire sauce

1 tsp mustard

Anchovy: ½ teaspoon

One tablespoon extra-virgin olive oil

You put the garlic in the food processor and process it. Put the mayonnaise, parmesan, lemon juice, worcestershire sauce, mustard, and anchovy (paste) in the food processor. Then drizzle in olive oil until it is combined. You can refrigerate this dressing for up to one week.

Herbed croutons

It makes 5 cups

Croutons aren't half the salad without tangy, creamy anchovies. These anchovies add crunch and creaminess to casseroles, egg dishes, and other dishes where a crispy topping is needed.

4 tablespoons (½ stick) unsalted butter, melted

2 tablespoons olive oil

1 teaspoon dried oregano. You are free to take some of those original words and rearrange them and repurpose them if

One teaspoon of garlic powder

½ teaspoon of salt A: The original is: The Market has Changed -- Inbound is the Response Your

¼ teaspoon cayenne

Preheat the oven to 350°F. Sprinkle the cubed bread in a large bowl.

In a bowl, combine the melted butter, olive oil, oregano, garlic powder, salt, and cayenne. Pour over cubed bread, and roll into balls. Toss the balls gently to help coat the bread.

Pour the cubes onto a sheet pan, in a single layer, and bake for 25 to 30 minutes, turning occasionally, until golden brown. Let the brittle cool on the pan, then transfer to an airtight container and keep in the refrigerator or cool pantry for up to 1 week.

Herbed croutons with extra virgin olive oil and parmesan

Makes 4 slices

A Caesar salad is served in restaurants all over the United States, and this garlic and lemon version is a top go-to. It's made sweeter using roasted red peppers as the dressing, giving it more flavor while staying healthful by avoiding oil and other added ingredients.

One pound of chopped romaine lettuce

¼ cup Garlicky Caesar Dressing

1/2 cup finely grated Parmesean cheese

1 Crouton

Salt and pepper

Transfer the romaine to a large bowl. Toss with the dressing.

Add the Parmesan cheese and breadcrumbs. Season with salt and pepper. Toss to blend.

Fried green tomato salad with garlic herb cheese and beans

Servings: 6

What do you do when your children wander into the garden and steal all the not-yet-ripe tomatoes? You create a new salad with fried green tomatoes, garlicky herb cheese, and a can of white beans. What makes this salad a restaurant specialty is it's presentation on a plate where the customer can eat the leftovers they just

A tablespoon of olive oil.

Try a balsamic vinegar dressing

1 teaspoon honey

¼ teaspoon of mustard (just dab it on) See also List of paraphrase External links Paraphrasing

A teaspoon of finely chopped fresh parsley

A small amount of minced garlic - 1-2 cloves

A serving of chicken contains ½ teaspoon salt.

1 (15-ounce) can of cooked white beans.

¼ cup finely diced red bell pepper

A cup of yellow cornmeal

The two servings of garlic powder

Just a pinch of ground black pepper

1 egg

1 tablespoon lukewarm water

One medium tomato, sliced 1/8 of an inch thick (16 slices)

Get the oil needed for frying ready

2+ tablespoons Garlicky Herbed Cheese

In a medium or large bowl, combine the olive oil, vinegar, honey, mustard, parsley, garlic, and salt to taste. Add the beans and red pepper, tossing to coat thoroughly. Set aside while you prepare the other ingredients.

This easy cornbread recipe includes garlic, pepper, and salt. To make the bread rise well, you should beat an egg with some buttermilk.

Use ½ of an inch vegetable oil in a large sauté pan or skillet over medium-high heat. Dip the tomato into the egg mixture, allowing the excess to drip off, and dust both sides of the tomato slice with the cornmeal.

Fry the tomato slices until golden brown on both sides. For each slice, fry about 3 to 4 minutes per side, until the slices become golden brown and start to get tender. Place the tomato slices on paper towels to drain.

To create a salad, put a fried tomato on a serving dish, then layer a few tomato slices that are sprinkled with cheese; spoon the bean dressing over the top of the salad and around the bottom of the tomatoes; and serve immediately.

Walnut and bean salad

Makes 8 to 10 servings.

This hearty salad is full of vitamins and minerals, but you get a great added value in taste with the walnut vinaigrette dressing. The toasted walnut oil is a tasty, nutty alternative to olive oil, and it adds a rich, nutty flavor to salad dressings. (Source

½ cup green beans, cut in half.

1 cup diced celery

½ cup diced red bell pepper.

1 (15-ounce) can whole, cooked red kidney beans, unsalted or regular

one 15.oz (400g) can chickpeas are drained, rinsed, and dried

150 grams (\about 7 ounces) of dried navy beans, rinsed, drained, and dried (\approximately 150 grams)

1/3 cup mixed seed oil

A ¼ cup red wine vinegar

½ Cup granulated sugar

A clove of minced garlic

1 tablespoon finely chopped fresh parsley

1/4 teaspoon salt

½ teaspoon of freshly ground black pepper

Bring a large pot of salted water, to a boil, over high heat. Add the green beans and a dash of black pepper and cook for 3-4 minutes, until tender. Remove from the water and place in a bowl of ice water to cool. After the beans are cool, remove them from the ice and place on a baking sheet covered with a clean dish towel to stop them

In a large mixing bowl, combine the celery, red onion, kidney beans, garbanzo beans, navy beans, and green beans.

In a large bowl, combine the dried black beans with the olive oil, vinegar, garlic, parsley, salt, and pepper; mix until thoroughly mixed. Refrigerate overnight prior to serving.

Roasted beet salad with goat cheese and candied nuts

Makes 4 to 6 servings

Cooking

This is the best salad you'll eat this season. You could never forget the salty cheese and crunchy walnuts when you're trying to remember this salad. The chopped beets taste like they've been roasted, while the

Beetroot that weighs about an ounce or 14 grams

½ cup walnuts halves

½ cup plus ½ teaspoon sugar is the best balance

A pinch of cayenne for a dash of heat

¾ cup white vinegar

1tbsp Dijon mustard

1 tablespoon of honey

1 tbsp. plus the rest extra-virgin olive oil

1/4 teaspoon Kosher salt

Use freshly ground black pepper

1 medium, sweet, yellow onion, cooked

¼ pound of crumbled goat cheese

Baby lettuce or baby spinach, sliced, for garnish

Preheat the oven to 350°F.

Wrap the beets in aluminum foil and bake for 1 1/2 hours or until a skewer inserted in the foil around the beet goes in easily.

While the beets are cooking, place the walnuts in a medium sauté pan. Pour water into the pan until the water is about half the diameter of the nuts and bring the temperature of the water up to medium-high. Continue to boil for 5 to 6 minutes, and then pour the nuts into a piece of foil to

Wash the beets and allow them to cool for about 30-40 minutes. To peel then, place them in cold water. You can use your fingers to remove the peel.

Place the beets in a large mixing bowl.

In a small bowl, combine the vinegar, mustard, honey, and oil. Whisk until the ingredients are blended. Season with salt and pepper, to taste.

Toss the beets with the dressing until they've been coated; then sprinkle the beets with caramelized onion, candied walnuts, and goat cheese; along with a nest of arugula.

Turkey lettuce tomato and bacon on a sandwich.

Make 4 servings

This is the salad version of a most popular sandwich, and it's so simple to assemble that once you find the right ingredients, this salad looks like it was baked. The dressing added a weight and substance to the salad that didn't give away that it

1 head lettuce, quartered

1 cup Hearty Blue Cheese Dressing or Buttermilk

1 cup diced tomato

1/4 cup chopped green onion

½ cup crumbled crisp-cooked bacon from (about) 8 strips of bacon

Pick up the head of lettuce by hand and remove the core with a large knife. Cut the head in half to produce 3 wedges. Place each wedge in a small bowl, drizzling each with ¼ cup dressing. Sift over each wedge 2 tablespoons tomatoes, 1 tablespoon green onion, and 2 tablespoons bacon. Serve as soon as possible.

Cherry walnut quinoa salad

Make it in batches of four.

With its growing recognition and popularity as a healthy food, people are experimenting with different ways to serve quinoa. Quinoa is not only a great source of protein; it provides a long list of essential nutrients and minerals. It also mixes well with many other foods.

1 cup couscous

Two cups water

One and a half cups' chopped broccoli florets.

1 cup dried cherries or cranberries

Finely chopped red onions

   cup chopped walnuts

¼ cup of white balsamic vinegar

Use 2 teaspoons of extra-virgin olive oil

30 whole cloves garlic, minced.

½ teaspoon salt

¼ teaspoon freshly-ground black pepper

In a medium saucepan, bring the Quinoa and water to a boil over high heat. The quinoa takes about 12-15 minutes to cook.

Turn the heat down to low, cover, and let simmer for about 10 to 15 minutes.

In large mixing bowl add cooked quinoa and allow to cool completely (to make eating easier later on).

In a large bowl, combine the broccoli, dried cherries, red onion, walnuts, and cooked quinoa.

In a small bowl, whisk together the 3 tablespoons of olive oil and the 4 teaspoon of sugar.

Add the quinoa mixture to the refrigerator overnight to let the flavors meld.

Fattoush

Makes 4 to 6 servings

My coworker, Chef Lisa first introduced me to this Lebanese salad made with toasted pita bread and seasonal vegetables and herbs; I loved it, so much that I took it one step further and created a gluten-free recipe. Food for Life Brown Rice Tortillas are the perfect substitute, so that everyone can enjoy it.

Two brown rice tortillas, each sliced

1-1-1

One teaspoon ground sumac

12 ounces cubed tomatoes

1/2-cup drained canned artichoke hearts

½ cup cubed cucumber

1 diced red bell pepper and ½ diced white bell pepper

½ cup diced red onion

5 radishes

2 tablespoons finely chopped fresh parsley

A spoonful of fresh mint

1 cup feta cheese

About a quarter cup roasted kalamata olives

Just ½ cup.

2 cloves of garlic

Coarse salt and freshly ground black pepper

Preheat the oven at 350 degrees (F).

First, toss the tortilla wedges in a bowl with 2 tablespoons olive oil and the sumac. Next place a pan in the oven; bake until crispy, 10 to 12 minutes. Lastly, take the tortilla wedges out of the oven and set them out on a plate.

In a large bowl, toss together the tomatoes, artichoke hearts, cucumber, red pepper, onion, radishes, parsley, mint, feta, and olives. In a small bowl, whisk together the remaining ¼ cup olive oil, the lemon juice, and the garlic. Pour over the salad and toss to coat. Season the salad with salt and pepper to taste and then mix in the crispy tortillas just before serving.

A recipe note: Sumac is one of the Middle Eastern spices found at any supermarket. It has a tart, fruity flavor – it can be used as a substitute.

The tangy grilled swordfish

Make 4 servings.

Marinade time: 4 hours

This citrus marinade is zesty with a nice punch, which makes it great for your favorite fish. Try it with swordfish, salmon, or mahi mahi.

Use 2 tablespoons gluten-free soy sauce.

2 tablespoons of freshly squeezed orange juice.

A tablespoon of ketchup

One tablespoon olive oil

1 tablespoon chopped parsley

2 pieces of garlic, chopped

1 teaspoon sesame oil

A teaspoon of freshly squeezed lemon juice

Use ¼ teaspoon oregano.

1/4 teaspoon freshly ground black pepper

A pinch of cayenne

1 lb of swordfish

Garnish with lemon and lime wedges

Put the soy sauce, orange juice, and ketchup in a medium bowl. Pour the olive oil over the soy sauce mixture. Mix with a fork, then add the parsley, garlic, sesame oil, lemon juice, oregano, pepper, and cayenne. Place the swordfish fillets in a large, resealable plastic bag. Pour the

Heat a grill to medium-high heat and preheat the grill. Grill the fish, on a piece of foil, for about 3 to 4 minutes, then turn the fish around and grill it 3 to 4 minutes more, until cooked to the desired doneness. Serve with a lemon and lime wedge.

Turkey and tart grape meat loaf

Makes about 6 servings

Cooking time: an average of 45 to 50 minutes

The green beans with cranberries and pork sausage complement the turkey and apples and enhance the flavor. When cooked, traditional meat loaves tend to be heavy on oil and meat with barely any vegetables or seasonings. They can be bland and dry.

1 tablespoon of olive oil

1 cup thinly sliced onions

5 cloves of garlic, minced

One large apple

Add ½ teaspoon dried thyme leaves to your food

2 pounds ground chicken

½ cup finely chopped dried parsley

½ cup light cream or half-and-half # How to make a paragraph paraphrase? A: I have a few

¼ cup salsa

2 teaspoons of gluten-free Worcester

2 eggs

1½ cups Italian-seasoned gluten-free bread crumbs

1 teaspoon of salt

½ teaspoon freshly ground black pepper

¼ cup of BBQ sauce

In a large bowl, mix together the wet ingredients and stir in melted butter.

In a heavy-bottomed pan, heat the olive oil. Add the onions and garlic and season. Let them cook, stirring, for 4 to 5 minutes to soften them then add the apple, thyme, and salt and pepper and let everything cook for another 2 minutes. Remove from the heat

Put everything in a bowl. Use your hands to mix all the ingredients and dish it up

Bake in a 9x5 loaf pan. Brush barbecue sauce on top, and bake for 45 minutes. Then, let it rest for 10 minutes and slice. Serve.

Chef note: If you cannot find apples smoked barbecue sauce, substitute your favorite barbecue sauce.

Creole sausage and shrimp with creamy biscuits and gravy

Yields 4 servings.

On a trip to New Orleans, I fell in love with the city's culture and its cuisine. The spicy shrimp is offset by the creamy grits, a combination typical of Creole cooking.

1 pound of shrimp, peeled and deveined

Season your food with ¼ to   can of Creole seasoning

A tablespoon of oil per day is best for your health

1 pound andouille sausage, diced

1 tablespoon butter

¼ cup of minced onions

1/4 cup of sliced celery.

¼ cup minced bell pepper

½ cup broth without gluten

½ cup canned diced tomatoes, drained

3 tablespoons of mustard

1 teaspoon cornstarch

Two tablespoons of light cream or half-and-half

Salt and pepper

Creamy Grits (recipe follows)

Let shrimp sit out until dry. In medium bowl, combine shrimp with Creole seasoning. Toss until completely coated. Set aside.

Heat some olive oil in a large skillet over medium-high heat; add the pepperoni or regular sausage and cook for 5 minutes, stirring often.

Add the shrimp to the pan, and cook for two to three minutes. Then, add the sausage, and let it rest.

In a large, heavy pan, melt the butter by cooking the onion, celery, and red pepper until tender. Whisk in the chicken broth, tomato sauce, Worcestershire sauce, and cream; add the sausage and shrimp. Simmer for a few minutes, until the flavors come together, then serve over hot grits.

Creamy grits

A few cups of gluten-free chicken broth

½ cup corn grits, gluten-free

2 tablespoons of cream

4 Tbsp (half a stick) cream

Salt and pepper

In a medium saucepan over medium-high heat, bring the chicken broth to a light boil. Let it sit until cold and then slowly stir in the corn grits, and cook until they thicken. Gradually add the cream and cook until fully reduced and thickened. Season with salt and pepper to taste.

Great walnut baked shrimp

For 6 to 8 people

Jumbo shrimp with a seafood stuffing made up of fresh crab, nuts, and crackers, and flavored with freshly crushed butter and white wine---delectable.

Crushed 1/2 cup walnuts

1 (4.4 ounce box) Glutino Crackers (about 32 crackers), crushed

6 teaspoons butter

2 tablespoons of celery.

¼ lb crabmeat

¼ cup wine

One pound (20 count) shrimp peeled and with tails on

In a large bowl, stir together the oats, almonds, honey and oats until blended.

In a medium sauté pan over medium-high heat, melt 3 tablespoons of the butter. Add the celery and allow it to cook for 90 seconds. Then add the remaining butter, crab, and white wine, and stir until the crab is cooked. Cool in refrigerator and stuff the mixture into the shrimp.

Put your oven to preheat to 400 degrees Fahrenheit.

Place some shrimp on a cooking sheet. Place 1 rounded tablespoon of stuffing on each shrimp. This makes a large amount of appetizer food for a small amount of time

Soft herb-crumbed scallops and mushrooms

Makes six to eight servings

My wife had our third child. This dish is so perfect for our family, so I've made it over and over again to please my children. I placed my buttery scallops on the stove and told my father-in-law to try a few bites before I'd add the recipe to the book. But just as the man was about to taste the appetizer, he turned to me and said, "When I met your

1.5-2 ounces lean steaks

1/4 teaspoon Kosher salt.

You should sprinkle pepper onto most of your food.

1/3 cup plus 1/2 cup melted butter

Minced garlic #

1 cup chopped mushrooms (about 3 ounces).

1 tablespoon apple cider vinegar

1¼ cup gluten-free bread crumbs

¼/cup finely ground gluten-free Glutino Paraphrase Crackers (about 2oz.)

2 tablespoons parsley

Add 1½ tablespoons of freshly squeezed lemon juice to your smoothie

Start preheating the oven to 400 degrees Fahrenheit and butter a 9-inch pie plate with a

Slice the scallops horizontally Place the slices in the crust dish Sprinkle the dish with the salt and pepper

Melt 3 tablespoons of butter in a large pan, add garlic and mushrooms, and cook, stirring, one minute. Then add sherry, cracker crumbs, and parsley and cook one minute.

Cover the scallops with the crumb topping, and with the remaining topping, sprinkle with some of the lemon juice, and cook for 12-15 minutes, until golden brown.

Gramma Nancy's stuffed peppers

Makes about 6 to 8 servings.

Cook it in one hour.

Giant sweet red peppers overflowing with a juicy mixture of ground beef, rice, tomatoes, and Parmesan and baked until hot and delicious, served with a salad and glass of red wine, make for a perfect comfort food meal for a cool fall night.

1 teaspoon salt

For each, cut a large red pepper lengthwise, with seeds

1 cup of long-grain brown rice

About 6 large tomatoes, chopped

25 grams finely chopped fresh parsley

¼ cup finely chopped basil leaves.

2 cloves chopped garlic

2 lbs ground beef

One cup diced green bell pepper

2/3 cup diced yellow onion

Add a teaspoon of kosher salt to each bowl.

Add ¼ teaspoon of freshly ground black pepper

¼ cup finely grated Parmesan cheese plus some extra for sprinkling

About 1/4 cup ketchup

1 tablespoon gluten-free Worcestershire sauce

Get the oven preheating to 350 °F. Oil your baking dish to ensure that the stuffed peppers cook evenly.

Add the salt to water in a pot. Bring to a boil, and add the red peppers. Cook for about 2 minutes, until the red peppers soften. Drain and set aside.

Cook the rice according to the directions.

With medium-size saucepan on medium-high heat, simmer the tomatoes, parsley, basil and garlic for between 15 to 20 minutes.

In a large skillet over medium heat, brown the meat, green pepper, onion, salt, and pepper. Then turn the heat down and let it simmer until the meat is evenly cooked through.

In a large bowl, combine the ground beef mix, tomato mix, cooked brown rice, ¼ cup of the parmesan cheese, ketchup, and Worcestershire sauce.

Arrange the peppers cut side up in a prepared baking dish and spoon a generous amount of filling into them. Sprinkle Parmesan cheese on top, and bake the peppers for 35 to 40 minutes, until heated through in the center. I'd be very grateful if anyone could check the paraphrasings

Pistachio-and-mustard-encrusted lamb chops

Make 4 to 6 servings...

These are ridiculously delicious. They taste like pistachios and a honey mustard glaze mixed with lamb meat. Use your porcelain and best cutlery to eat them like a lamb chop appetizer.

1½ pounds of a frenched, cut and divided rack of lamb

Salt and peppers.

1 teaspoon of olive oil

3 teaspoons of mustard

2 cloves of garlic

Half cup dry-roasted pistachios

1 Tablespoon of cornstarch

Preheat the oven to 400°F while greasing a baking sheet.

Sprinkle the lamb chops lightly with salt and pepper.

Heat olive oil in a skillet and pan-sear the pork chops for 1 minute each side. Place on the oiled pan to dry.

Put two of them together in a bowl and mix them up.

Using a food processor, mix the pistachios, a pinch of salt and pepper, cornstarch and 1 tablespoon of mustard together. Spread a layer of mustard on the inside of each chop and press it into the mixture to ensure that the chop gets coated. Then place the chops on a baking pan so the crust comes up. Bake the chops for 10 minutes at an external temperature of 145°F. Serve right away.

Apple barbecued ribs

Makes enough to serve 6 to 8

Marinating time: Overnights & a

Cook time 4 ½ hours

This hot pepper sauce makes for succulent, mouth-watering, finger-licking-good baby back ribs.

Dry Rub (recipe)

6 lb baby back pork ribs

Plum Sauce

Put on your hands, massage the dry rub over the ribs, until it is all coated evenly. Cover the ribs, and refrigerate overnight.

Preheat the oven to 200 degrees Fahrenheit and line a baking sheet with aluminum foil.

Put the ribs on a rack to let sit on the lined cookie pan and let them cool. Heat a grill, turn the heat to medium, and let the grill be hot.

Apply the plum sauce to the ribs, and cover with foil, cooking for 30 minutes. Remove and brush with plum sauce. Flip the ribs and brush with more sauce. Cover and cook another 10 minutes.

Dry rub (makes about ¾ cup)

Put 3 tablespoons of ground allspice

2 tablespoons brown sugar

3 tablespoons of garlic powder

1 tablespoon of kosher salt

1/2 teaspoon freshly-ground nutmeg

1 teaspoon of ground cinnamon

1 teaspoon dried basil leaves

1 teaspoon of dry mustard

In a medium mixing bowl, combine all the dry rub ingredients. Combine well. The mix can be stored loosely sealed in the refrigerator for up to 4 weeks.

Put 1½ cups of the ingredients in a food processor and blend until smooth.

½ cup raspberry jam

½ cup rice vinegar

½ cup of relish

¼ cup of honey

1 tablespoon minced garlic

¼ cup freshly squeezed lime juice for 30-60 seconds

1-tbsp chopped sweet onion

½ cup plum wine

In a large pan over medium heat, combine the plum wine, vinegar, ketchup, honey, garlic, lime juice, and onion and let the sauce simmer for 5 minutes. Add the plum wine and let the sauce simmer for 5 minutes. Remove from the heat and allow the sauce to cool at room temperature. Refrigerate the sauce if it is being made ahead of time. It will keep for up to 1 week.

CPSIA information can be obtained
at www.ICGtesting.com
Printed in the USA
LVHW061928190722
723838LV00007B/46